femalia

Joani Blank, Editor

Photographs by

Tee A. Corinne
Michael Perry
Jill Posener
Michael A. Rosen

Down There Press
San Francisco

Library of Congress Cataloging-in-Publication Data

Femalia / Joani Blank, editor : photographs by Tee A. Corinne ... [et al.].
p. cm.
Includes bibliographical references.
ISBN 0-940208-15-6 (pb) : $14.50
1. Vulva—Anatomy—Atlases. I. Corinne, Tee, 1943-
QM421.F45 1993
611'.67—dc20 93-2328
CIP

We also offer librarians an Alternative CIP prepared by Sanford Berman, Head Cataloger at Hennepin County Library, Edina, MN, which may more fully reflect this book's scope and content.

Alternative Cataloging-in-Publication Data

Blank, Joani, 1937- editor.
Femalia, Joani Blank, editor. Photographs by Tee A. Corinne, Michael Perry, Jill Posener, and Michael A. Rosen. San Francisco, CA: Down There Press, copyright 1993.
"Thirty-two full-color photographs of women's genitals... The vulvas...belong to a group of women diverse in age, race and ethnicity."
Includes bibliography.
1. Vulva—Pictorial works. 2. Erotic photography. 3. Photography of women. I. Title. II. Title: Female genitalia. III. Down There Press. IV. Corinne, Tee A., illus. V. Perry, Michael, illus. VI. Posener, Jill, illus. VII. Rosen, Michael A., illus.
611.67 or 778.924 or 778.928

Additional copies of this book are available at or your local bookstore or directly from the publisher:
Down There Press, 938 Howard Street, #101, San Francisco CA 94103
Please enclose $18.00 for each copy ordered, which includes $3.50 postage and handling.

Printed in Hong Kong
9 8 7 6 5 4 3 2 1

INTRODUCTION

Almost sixteen years have elapsed since I published *I Am My Lover,* a book of photographs of women masturbating, with sixteen color portraits of women's genitals in two "centerfolds." That was at the height of the women's self-help movement, when in clinics around the country a few women were fortunate enough to view and examine their own genitals and those of other women, in many cases for the very first time. Except for this tiny minority of the adult female population, most women then had virtually no way of knowing what other women's genitals looked like.

Some might wonder how such knowledge benefits women. My many years of doing sex therapy and leading women's sexuality workshops have taught me that without such information a majority of women believe to this day that, in one way or another, their genitals are not quite "normal."

With the publication of Betty Dodson's *Liberating Masturbation* (now out of print) and Tee Corinne's *Cunt Coloring Book* in the seventies, women finally had some images of other women's genitals to refer to, but these were drawings, not photographs. The artistry of these drawings was acknowledged and widely appreciated by women and men alike, and the liberating quality of the images was rightfully touted by feminists of various stripes. Still, outside of "men's" magazines, where the women's genitals were often powdered and half-hidden, and the images often modified and airbrushed, women had no resource for photographic representations of vulvas. Remarkably, that state of affairs has not essentially changed until the publication of this volume.

That speaks to the sexual consciousness-raising of these pictures. But what about their erotic potential? These are pictures of genitals, and for that reason alone they will be interesting to most people, interesting and beautiful to some, and interesting, beautiful and arousing to others. To encourage your direct connection with the pictures, I have chosen to publish them one by one and, aside from this brief introduction, without words.

The vulvas pictured here belong to a group of women diverse in age, race and ethnicity. Some have experienced childbirth. There is also variation in style, color, size and proportion. Like faces, these genitals all have the same parts in essentially the same arrangement, and we have included a labeled drawing for those who may find a "map" helpful.

None of these women was sexually aroused at the time her vulva was photographed. When a woman is aroused, typically her clitoris enlarges, her labia become noticeably engorged, and vaginal lubrication increases. The vulva may change in appearance during a woman's menstrual cycle as well.

Several of the women whose genitals are pictured here have shaved some or all of their pubic hair, and two have had their labia pierced with jewelry. Both shaving and the wearing of jewelry are primarily done for aesthetic reasons, although women who shave their outer labia generally report that they enjoy the heightened sensitivity of the bare skin. If you find the photographs of pierced genitals disturbing, it may reassure you to know that piercings of the labia or clitoral hood hurt less and heal considerably faster than pierced ears.

I am pleased to call each of the four photographers whose

work is represented here friends. Tee A. Corinne and Michael Perry did most of their genital portraits many years ago and were pioneers whose slides have been used in hundreds of human sexuality college courses. Many of Tee's pictures graced the pages of the original *I Am My Lover*. Professional photographers Jill Posener and Michael A. Rosen took the photographs included here specifically for this book. Although both have done sexual photography, neither had taken closeups of this kind before. I am mightily grateful to all four of these talented artists for their contributions to this project.

I found the word "femalia" in Nicholson Baker's delightful short novel, *Vox*. Thanks, Nick, for solving the what-shall-we-name-the-book problem for me.

Learn from these photographs, appreciate their beauty, allow them to give you pleasure.

Joani Blank
June 1993

Portfolio I, Photographs by Tee A. Corinne ➤

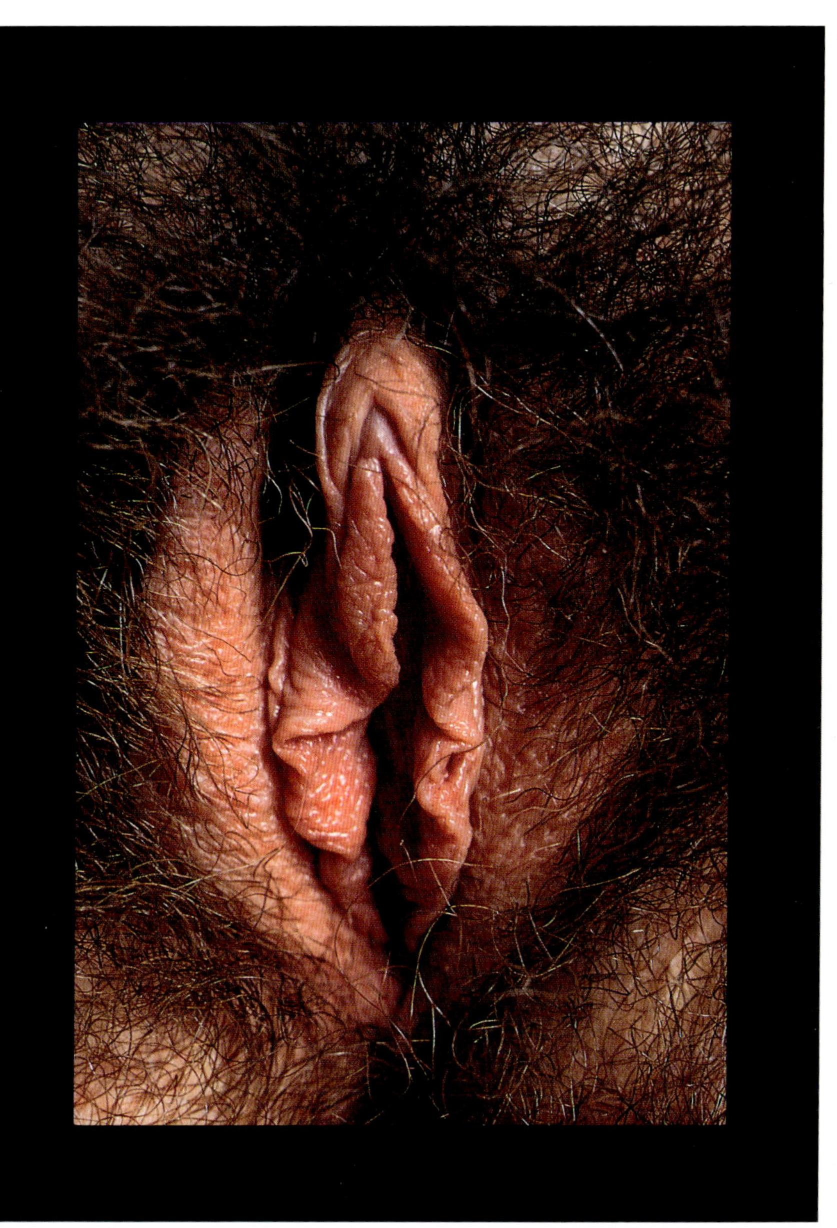

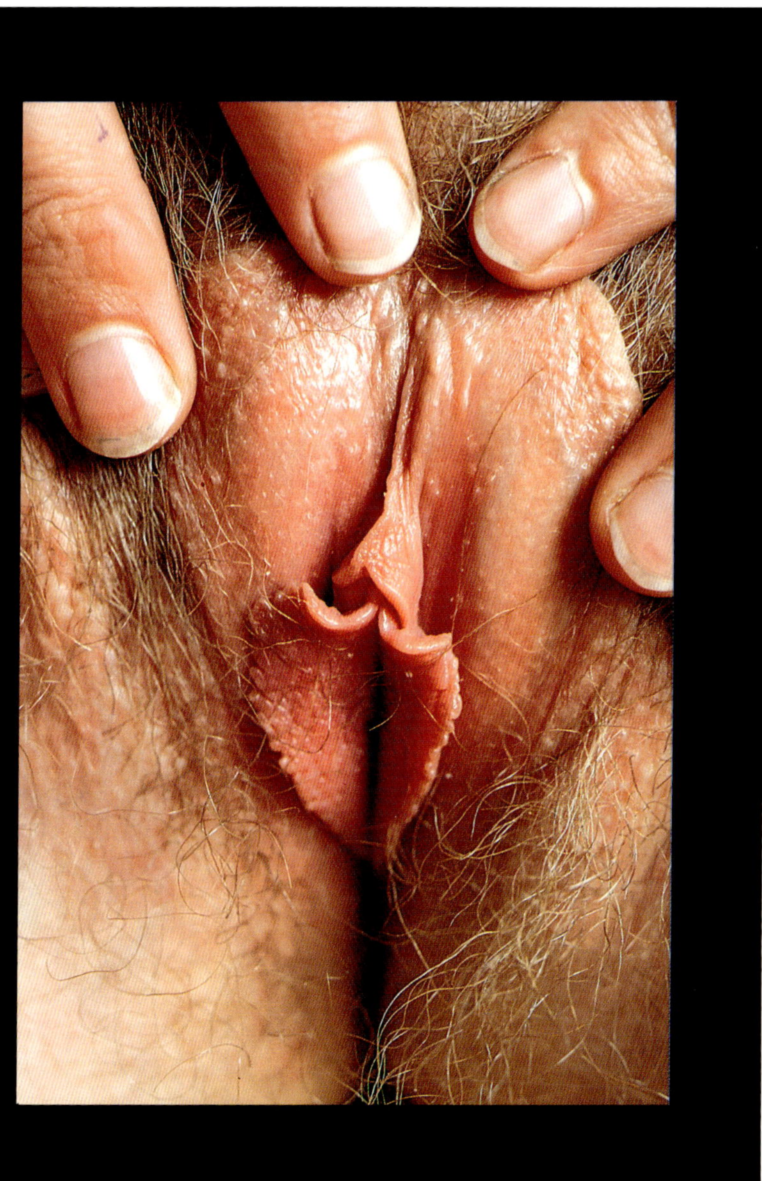

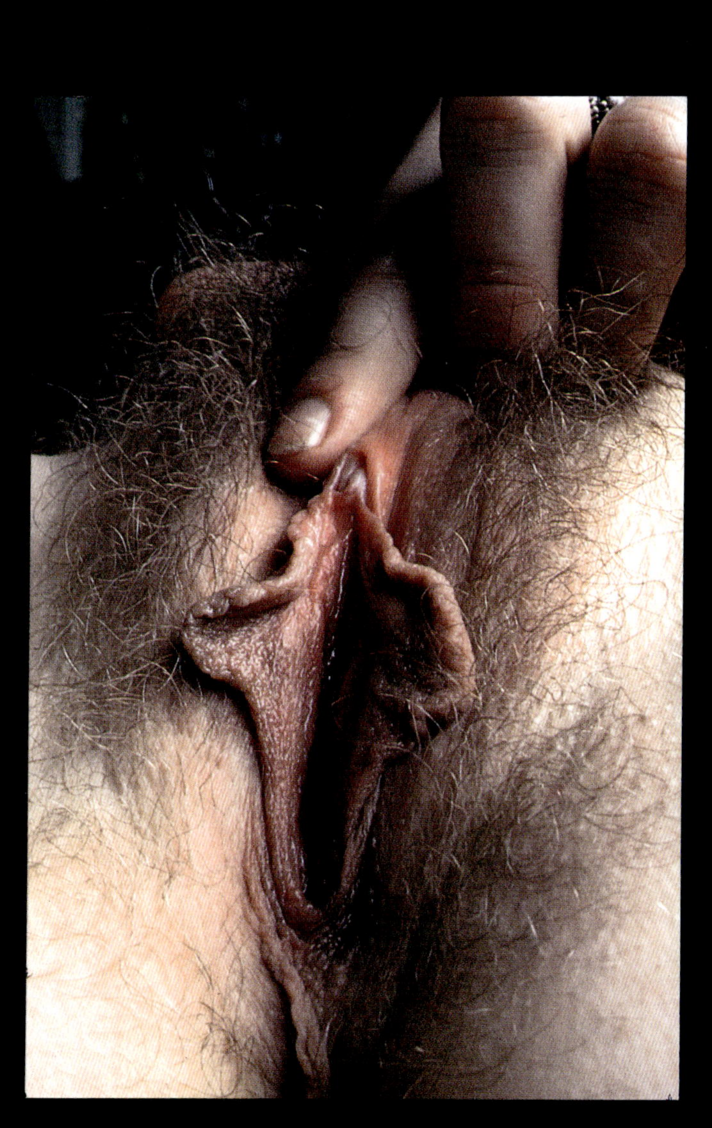

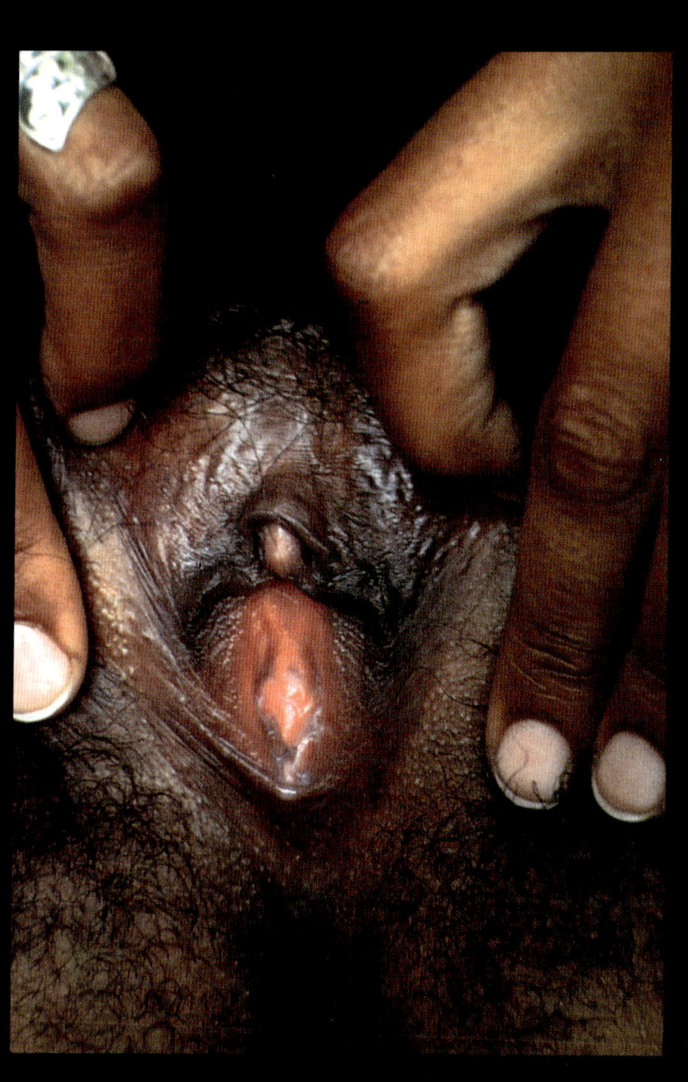

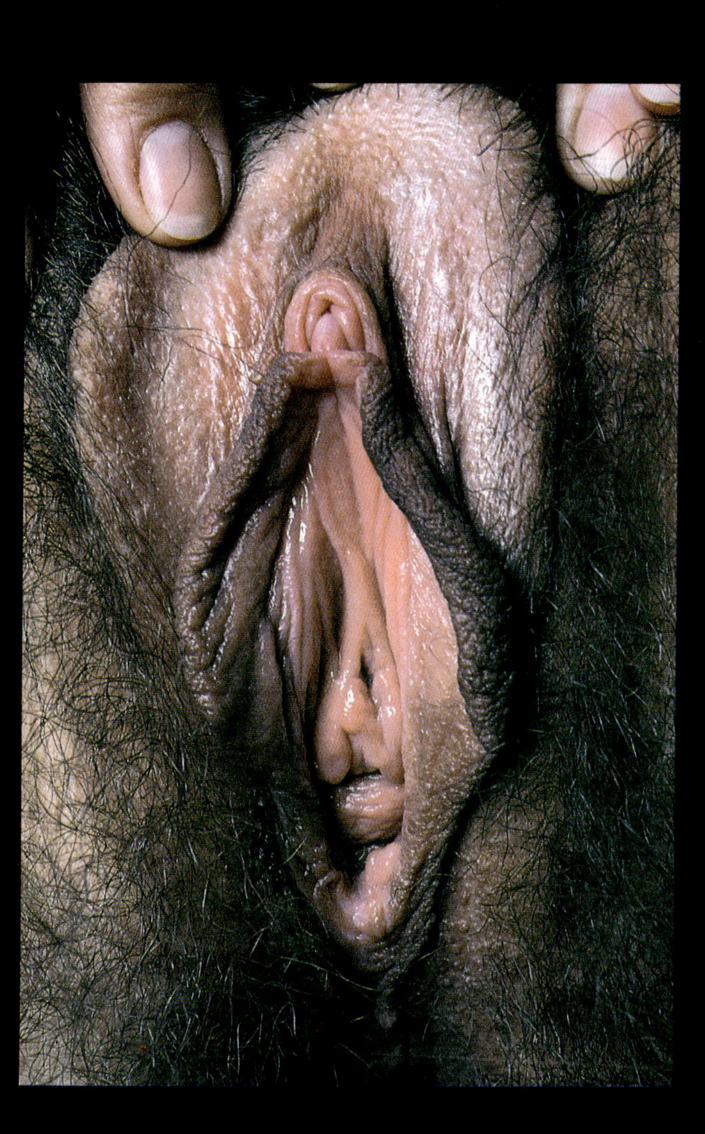

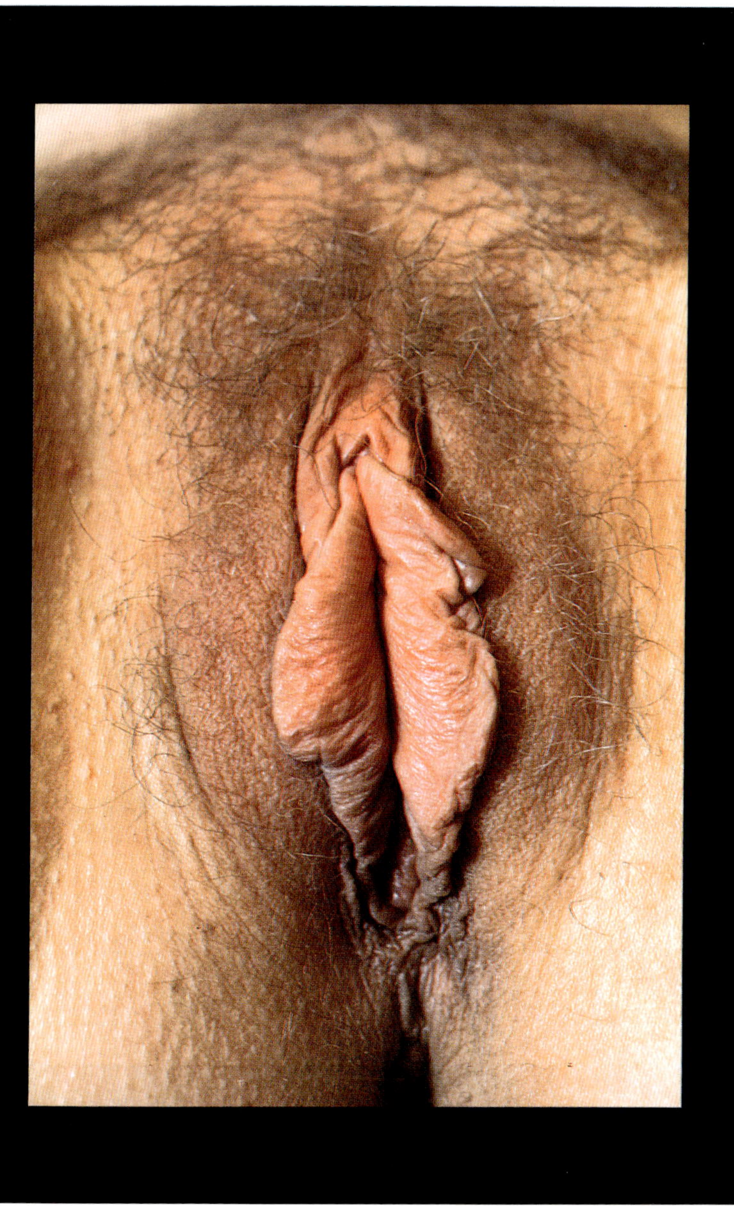

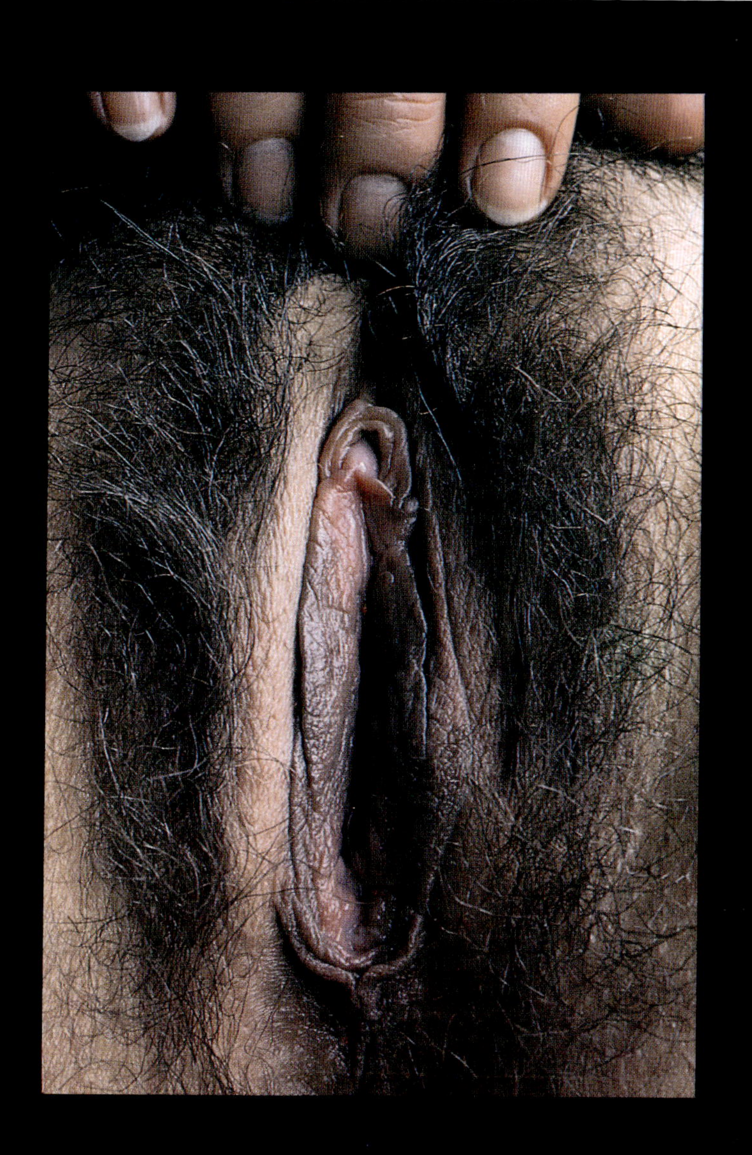

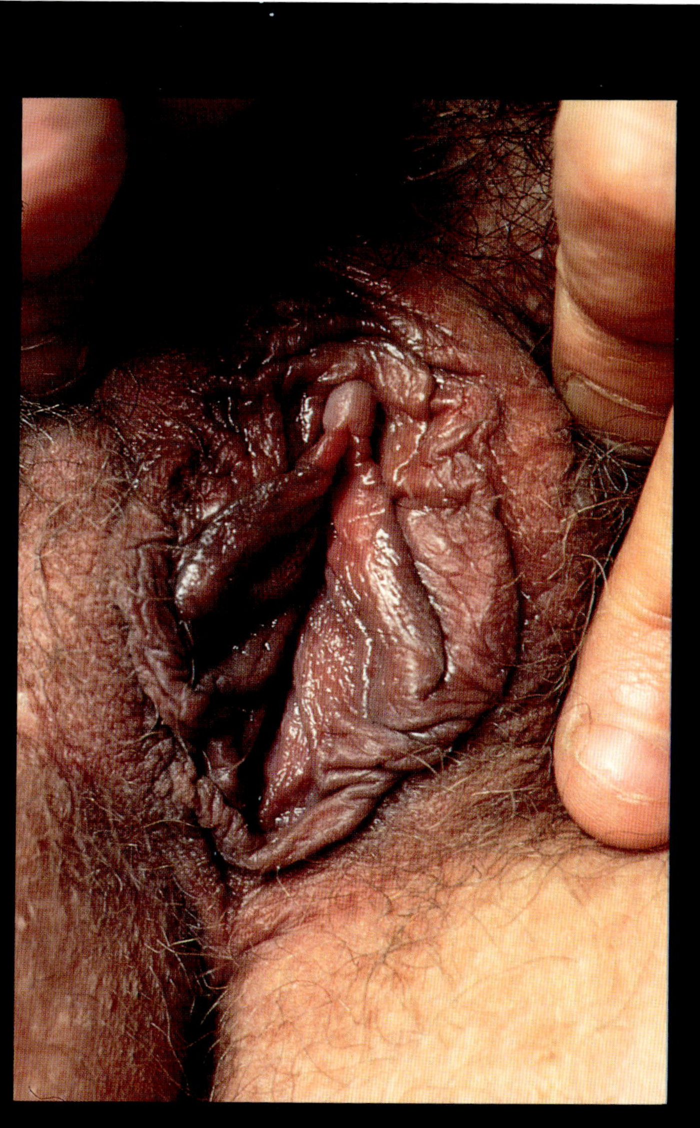

Portfolio II, Photographs by Michael A. Rosen ➤

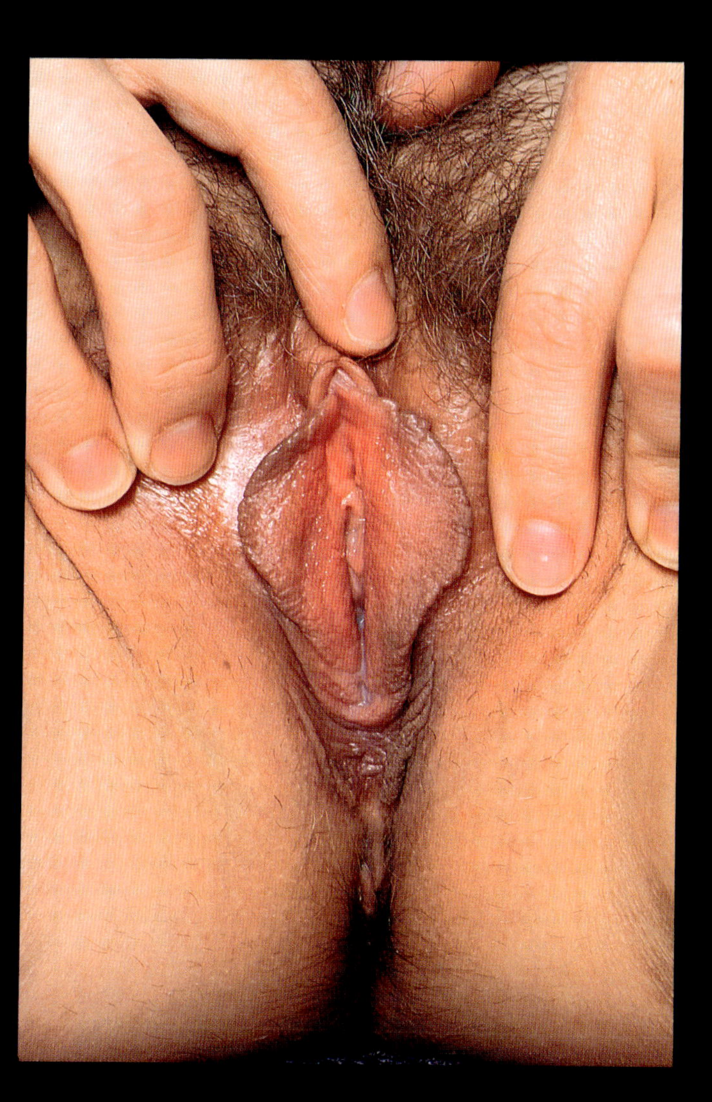

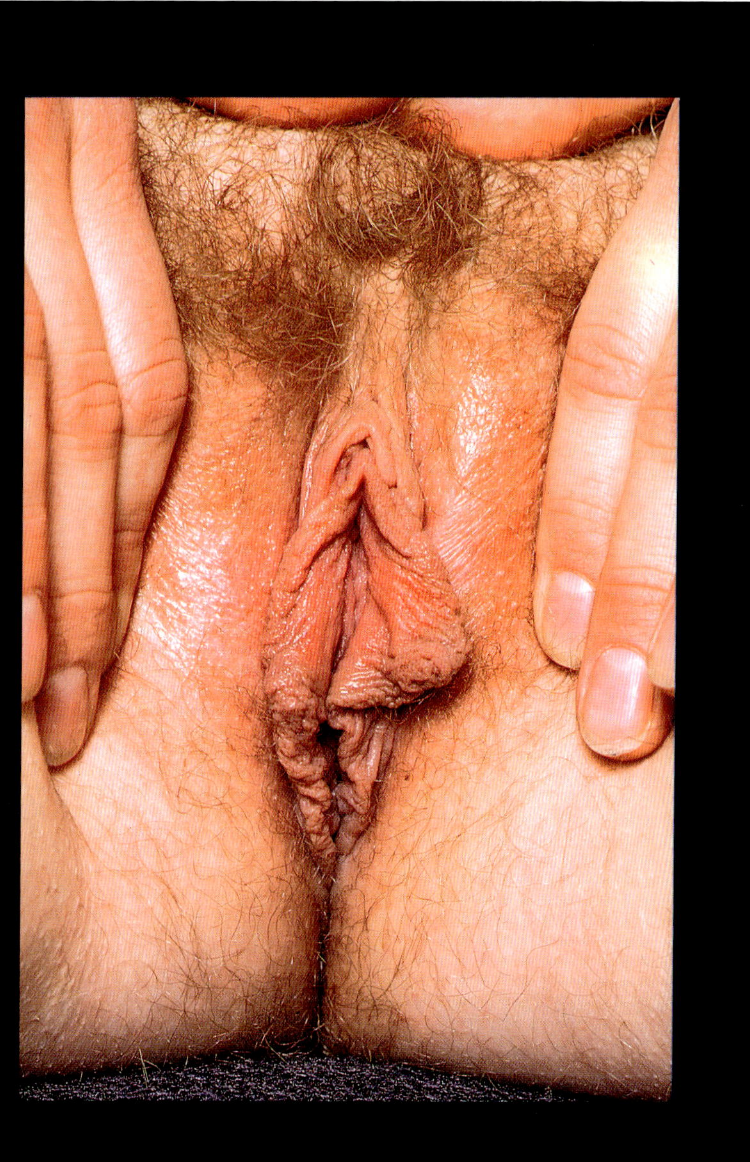

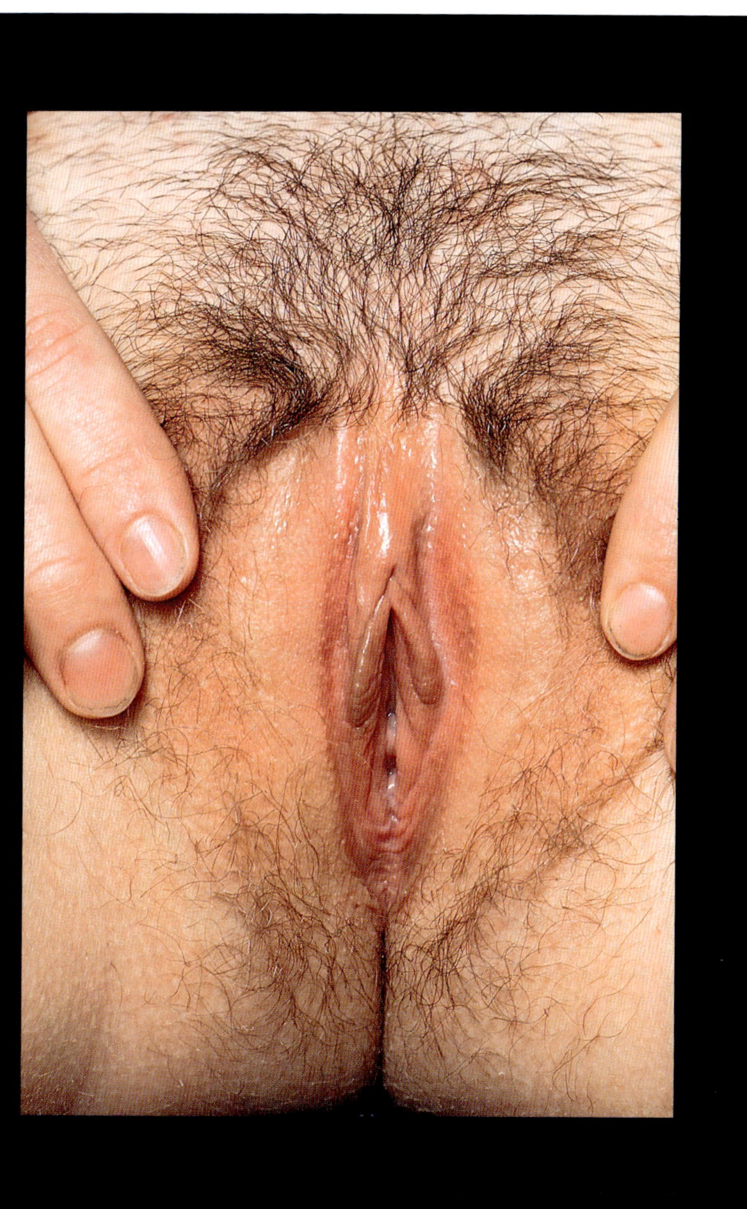

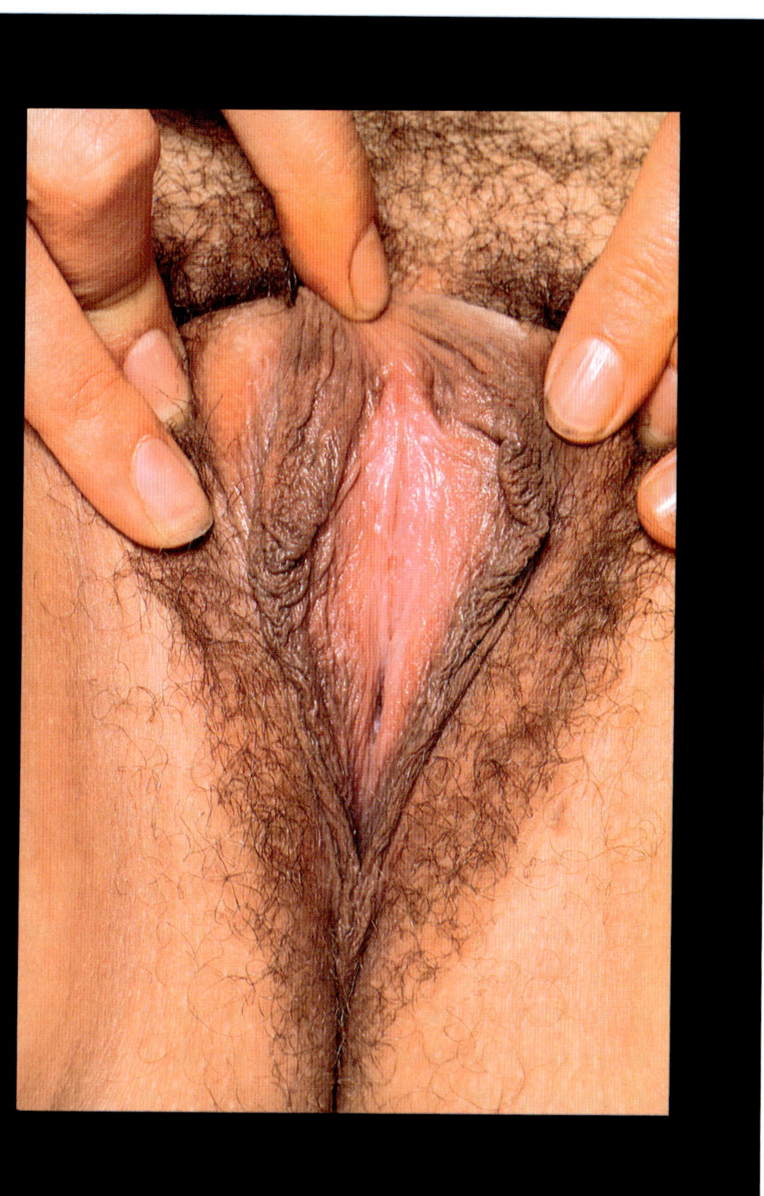

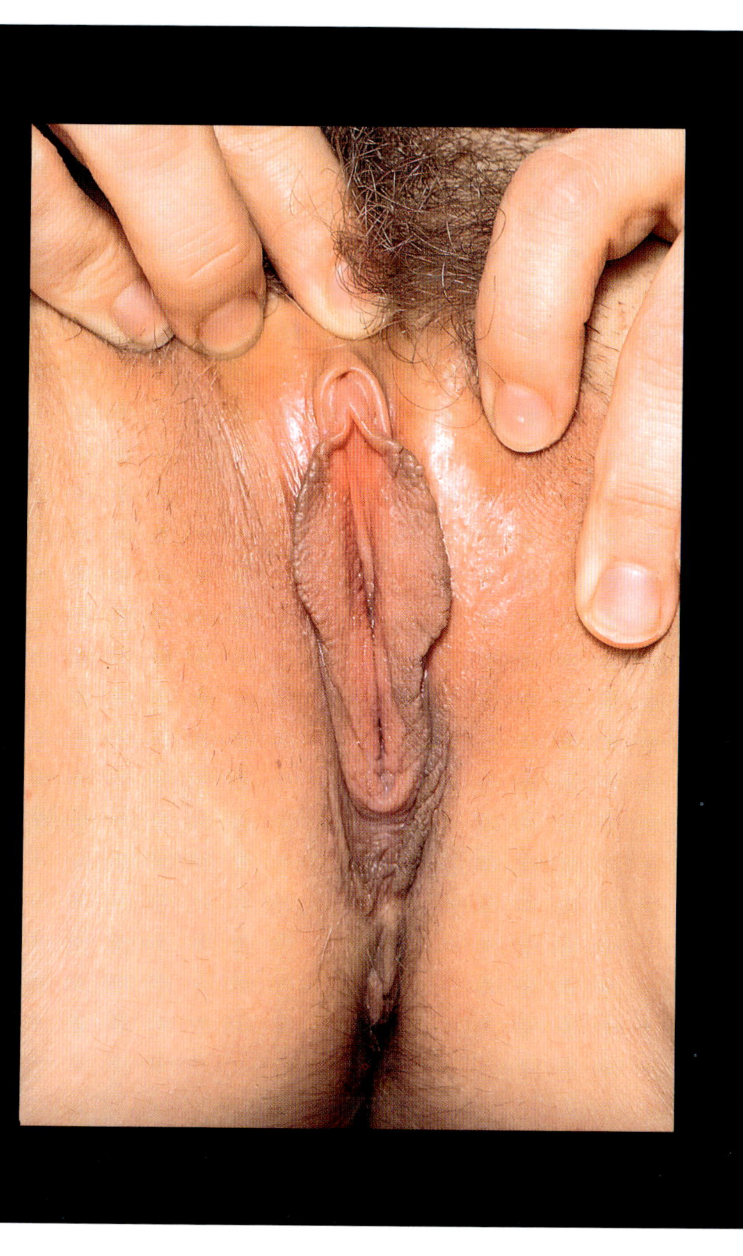

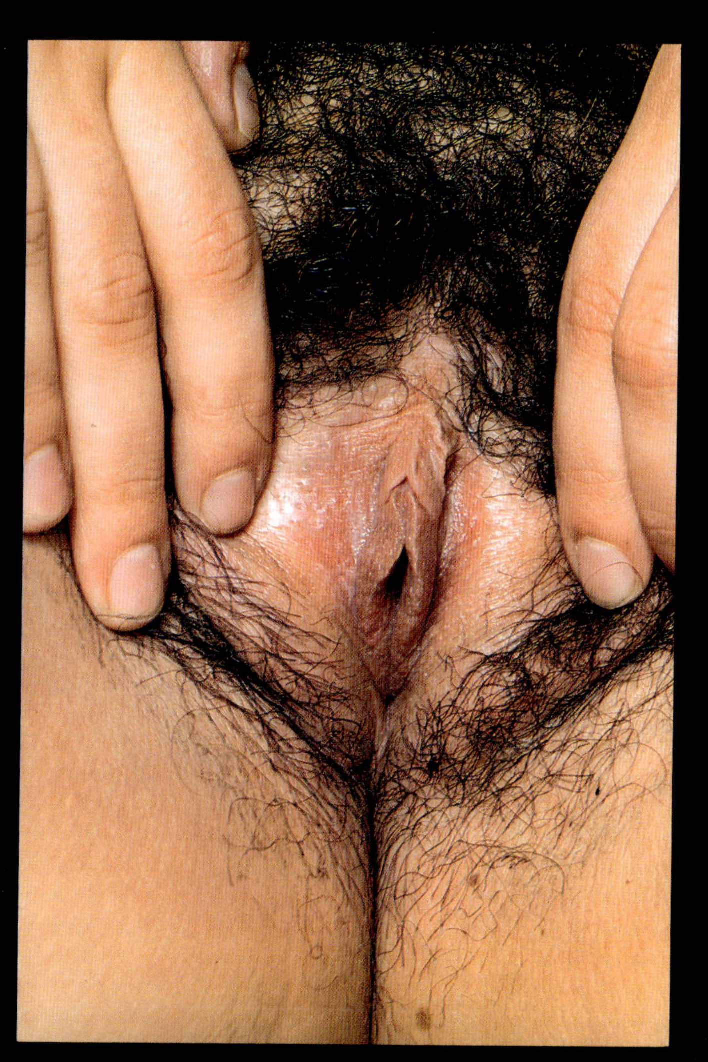

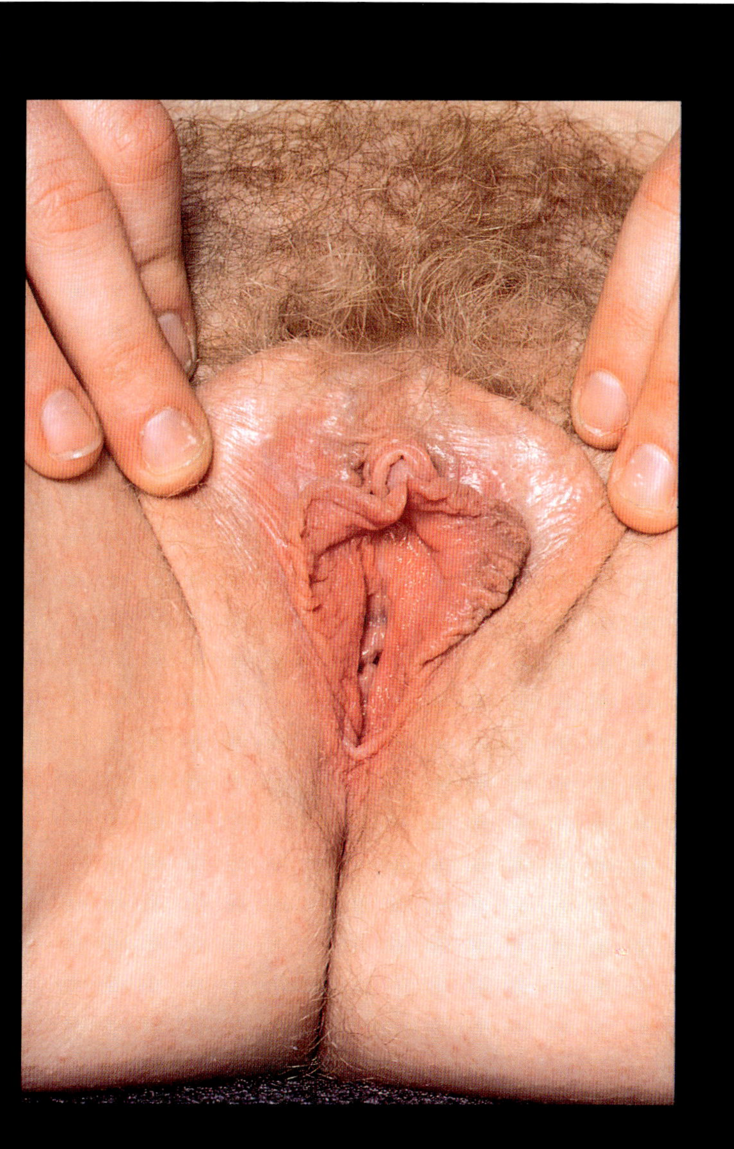

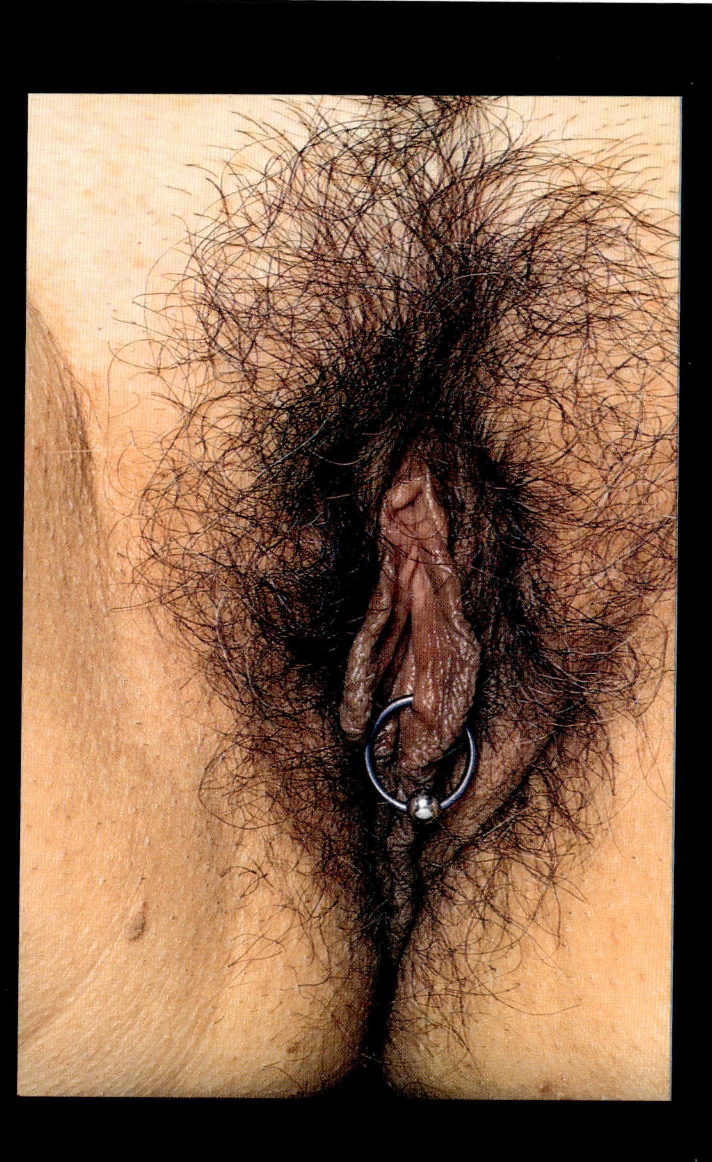

Portfolio III, Photographs by Jill Posener ➤

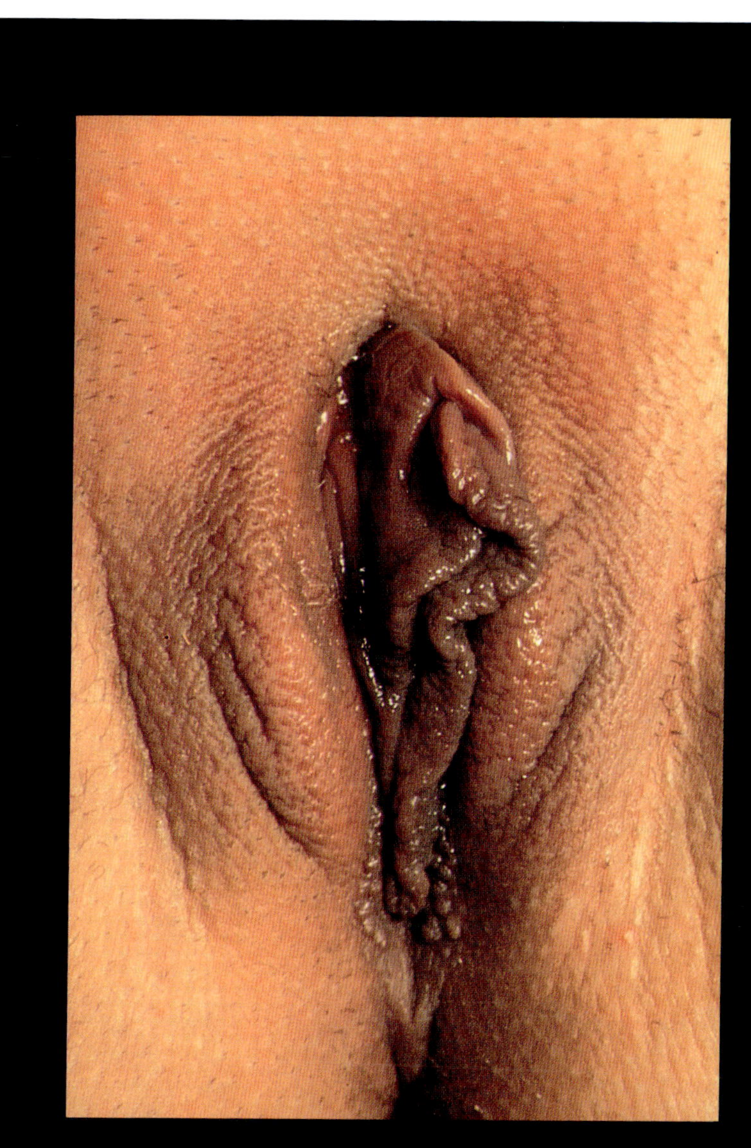

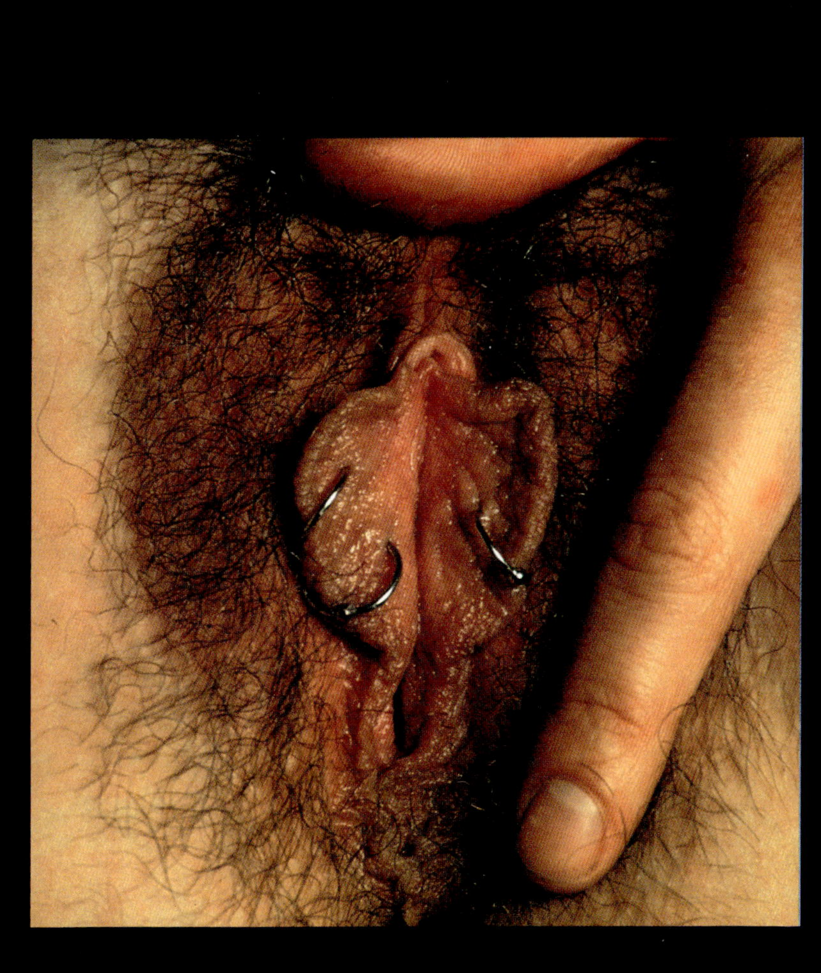

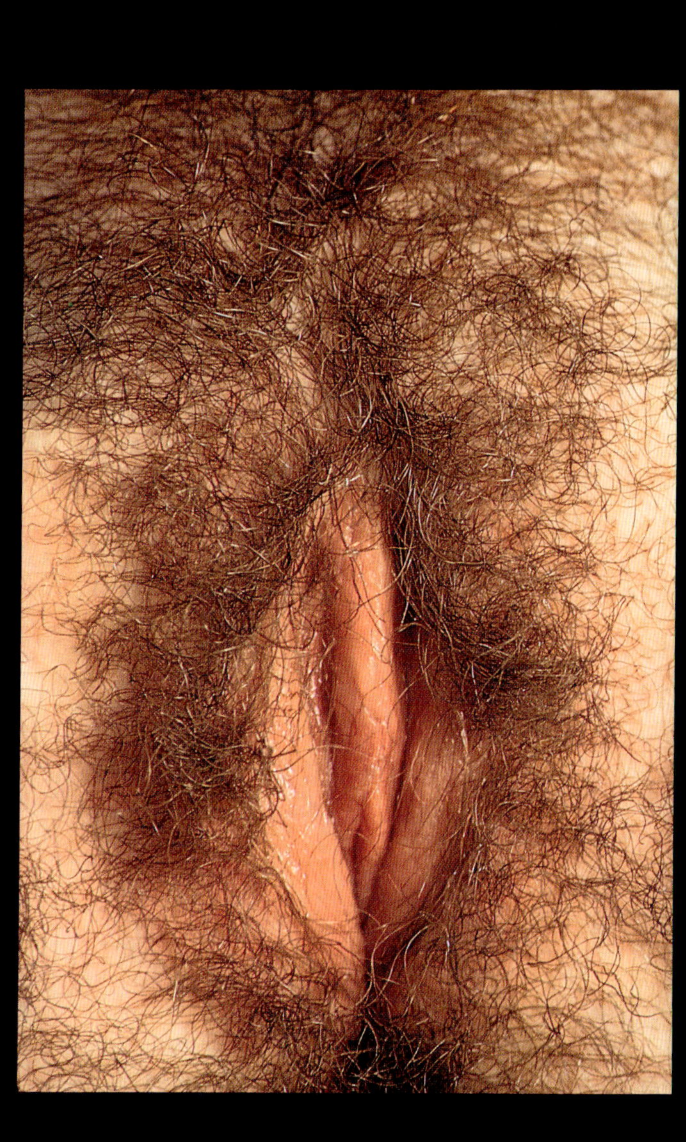

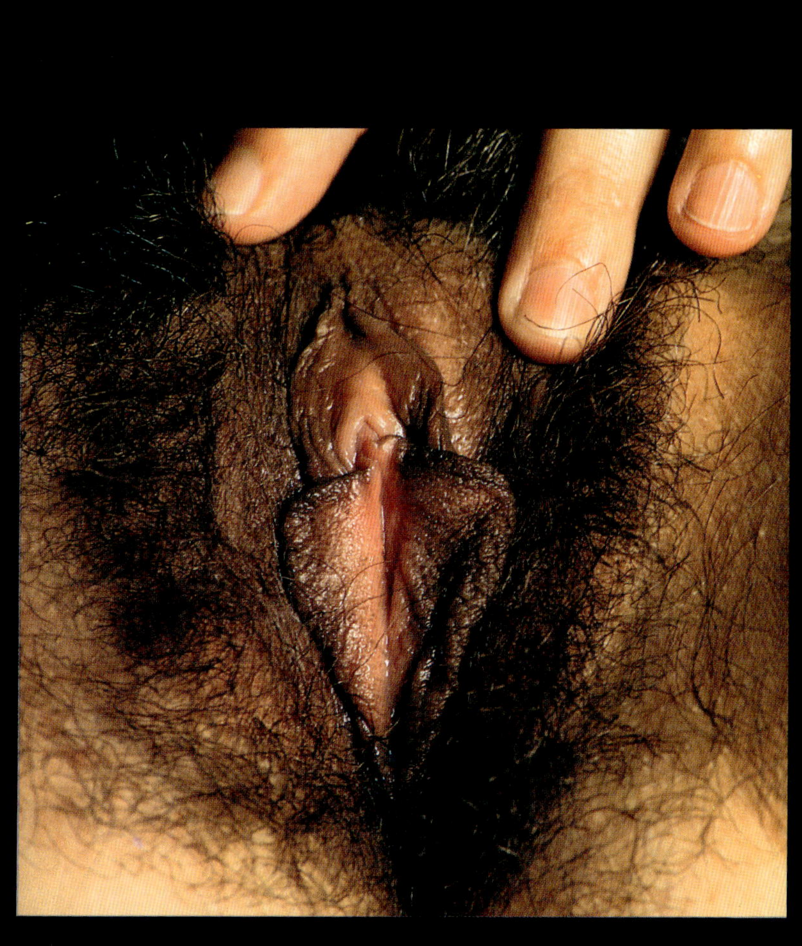

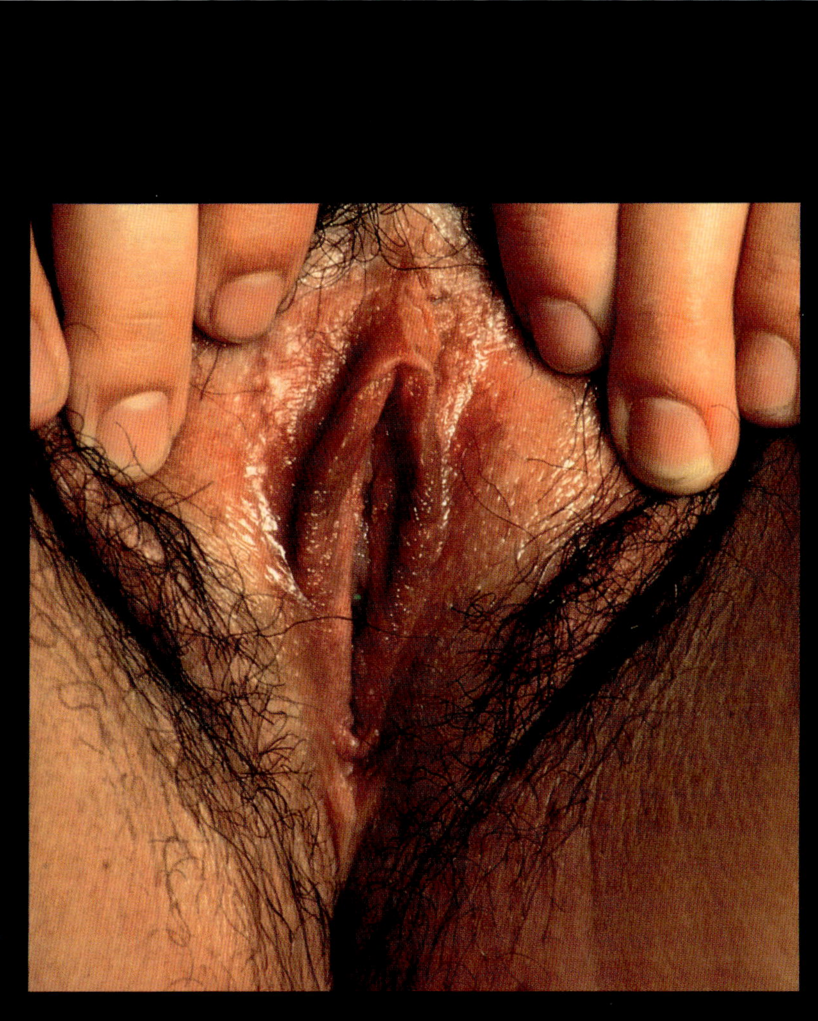

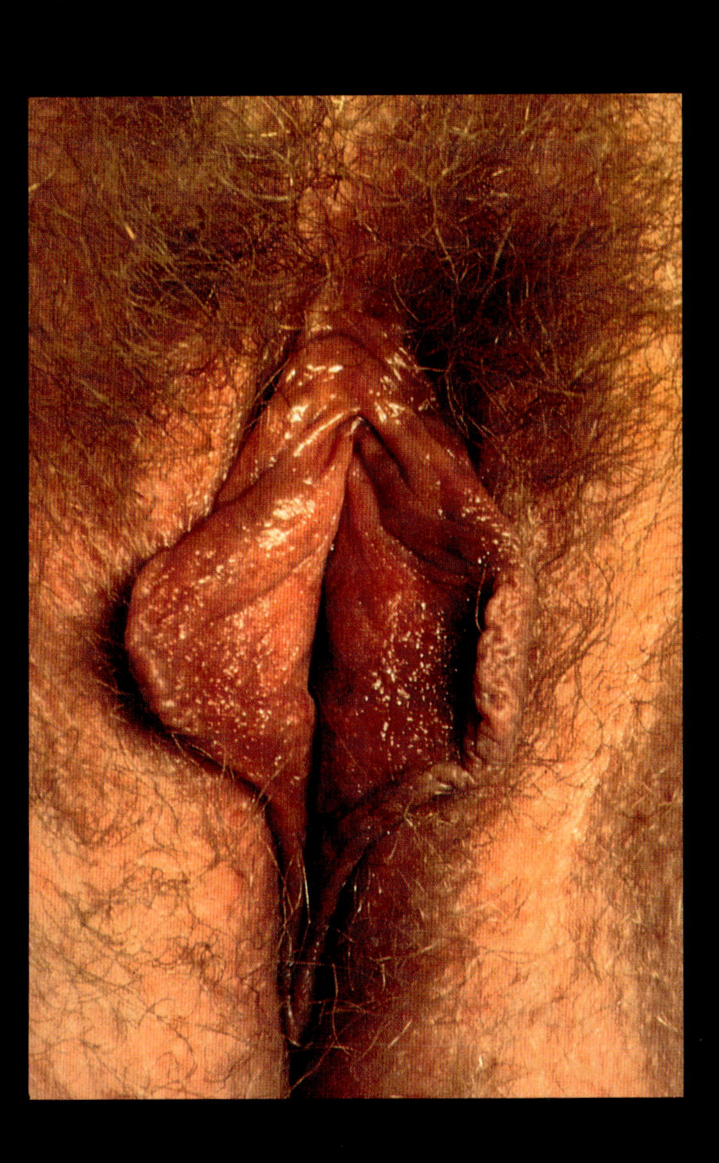

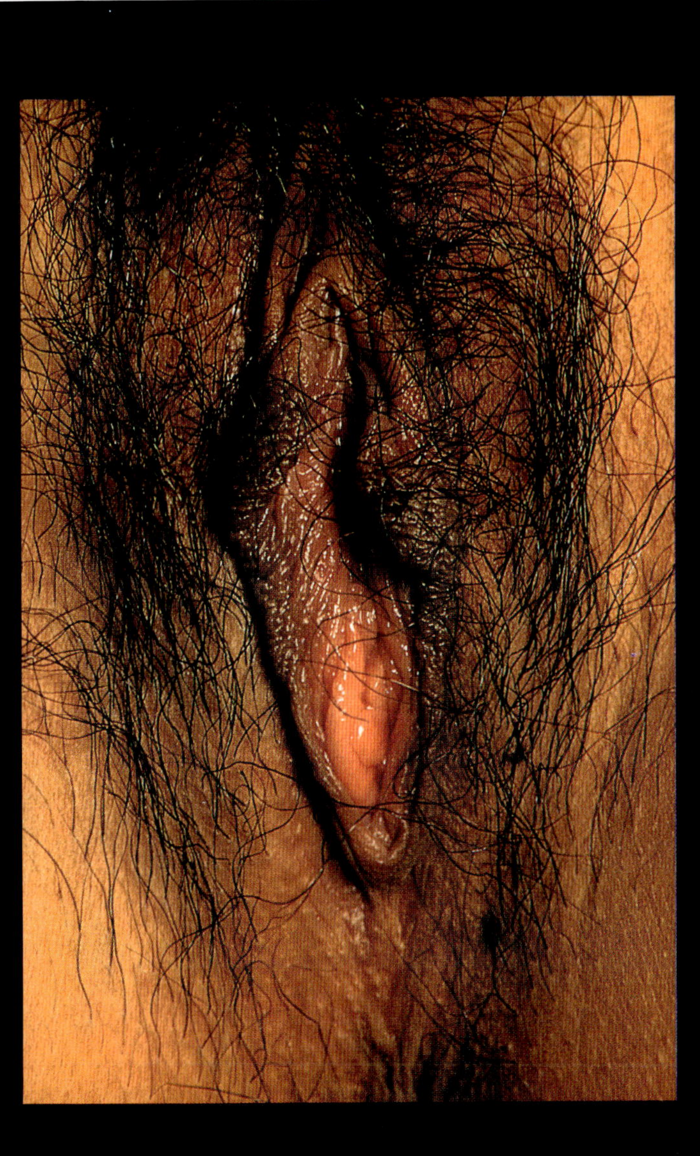

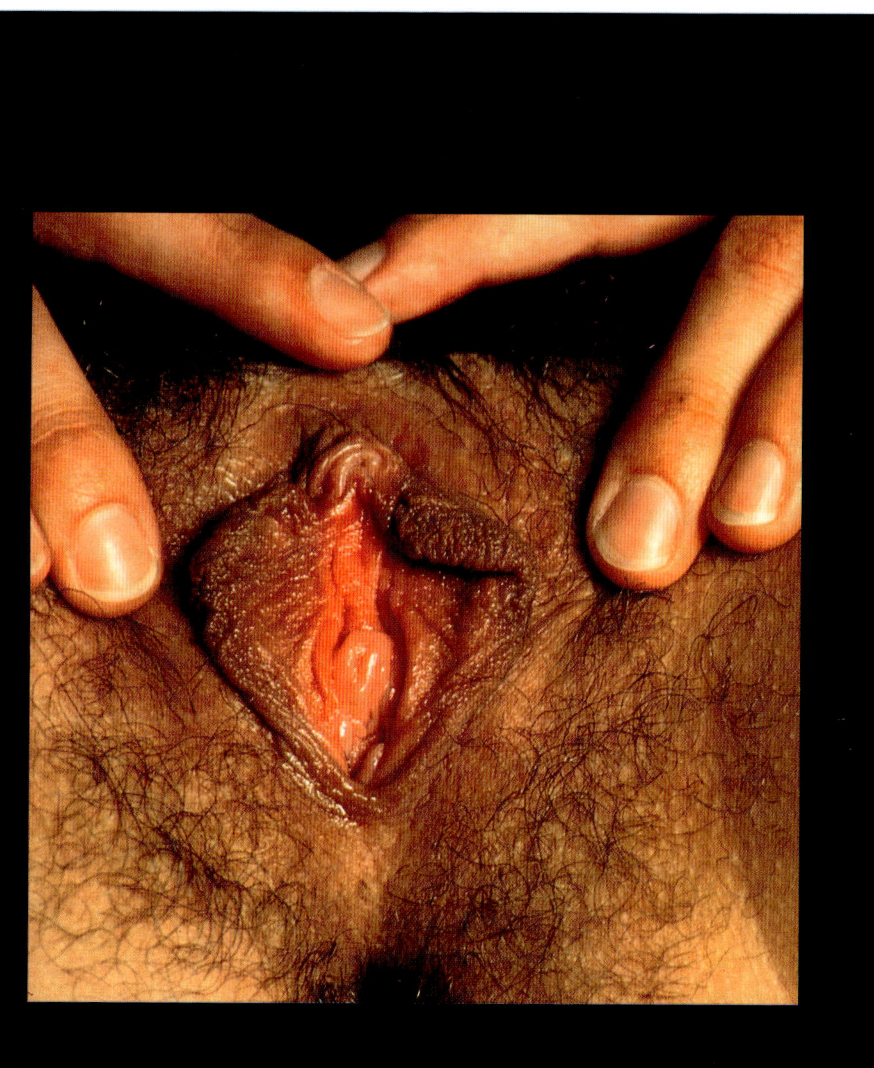

Portfolio IV, Photographs by Michael Perry ➤

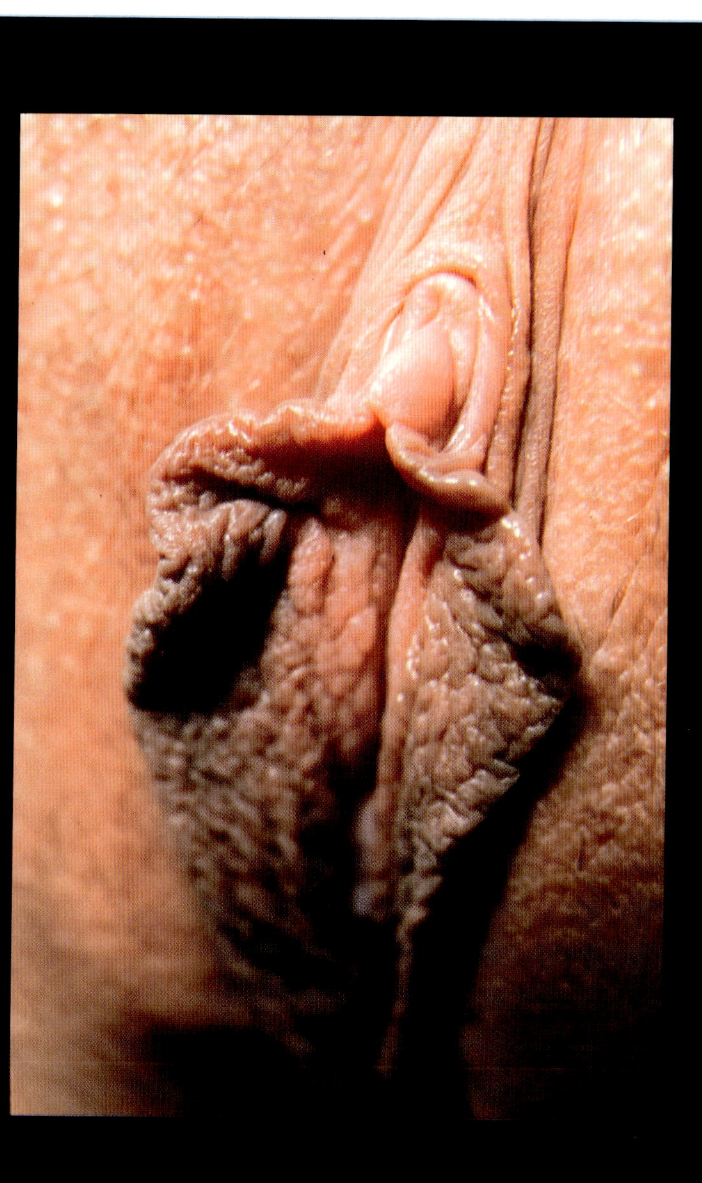

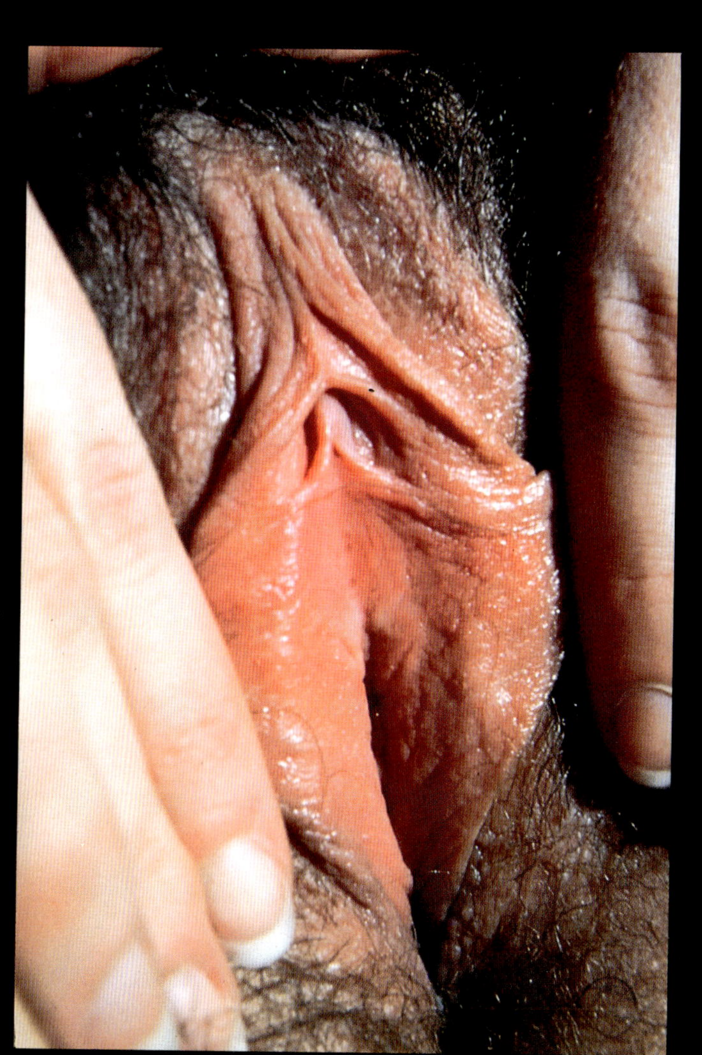

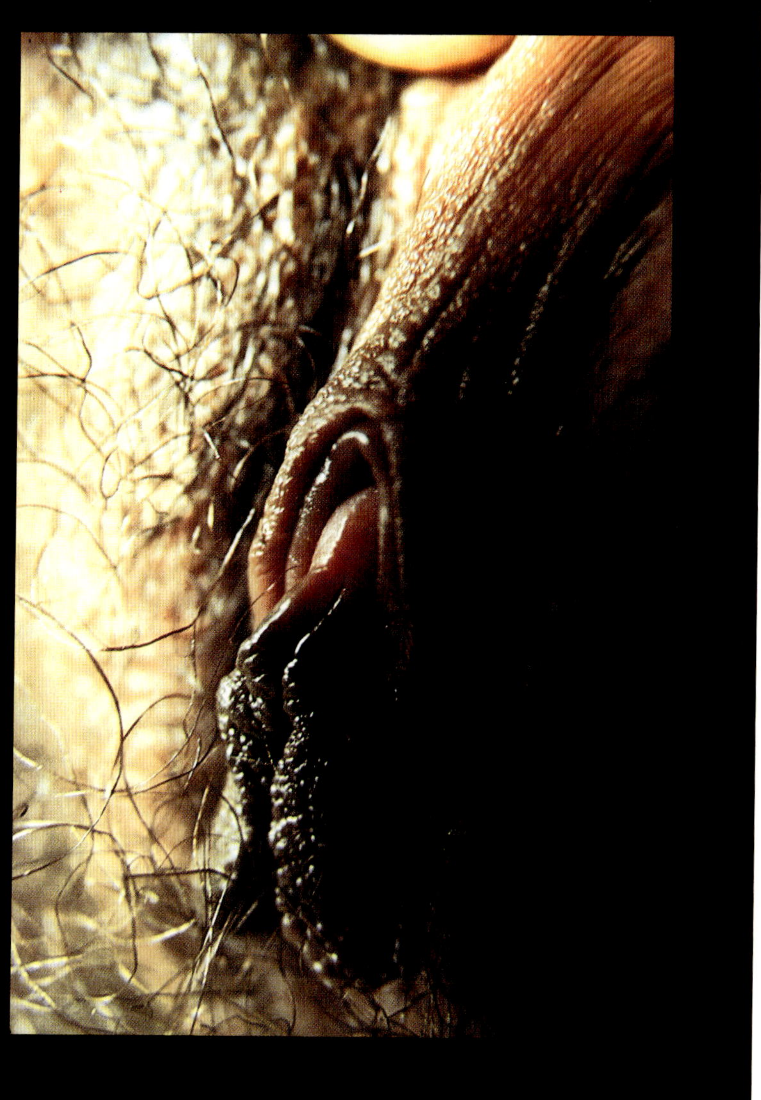

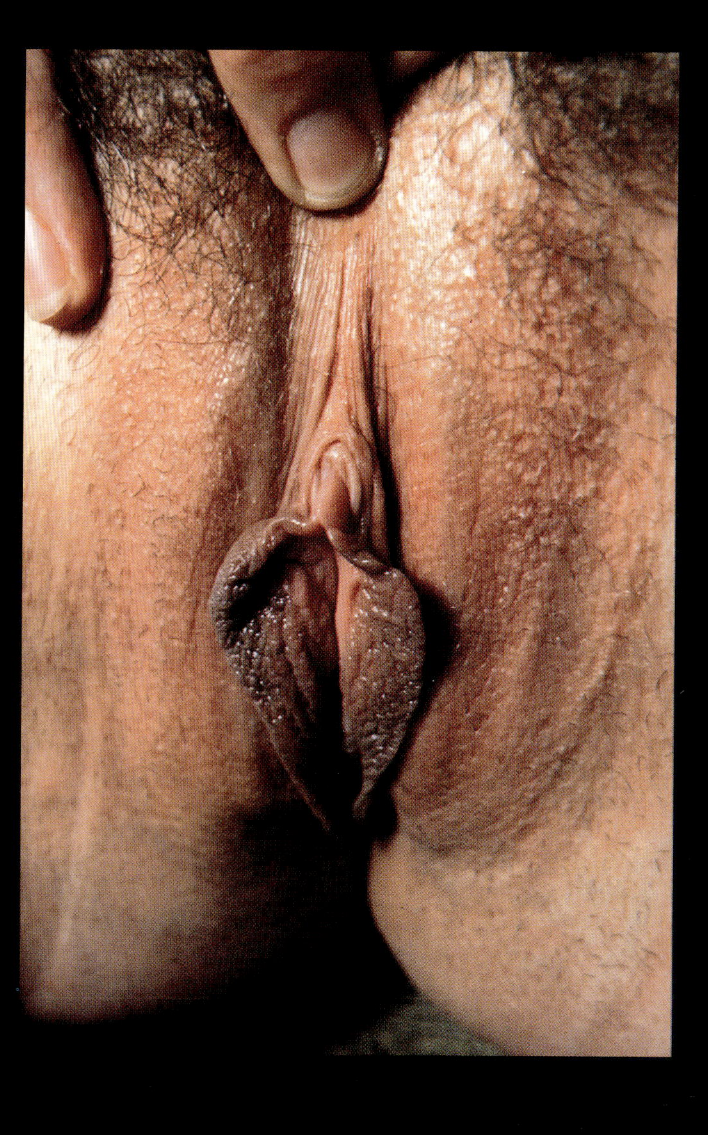

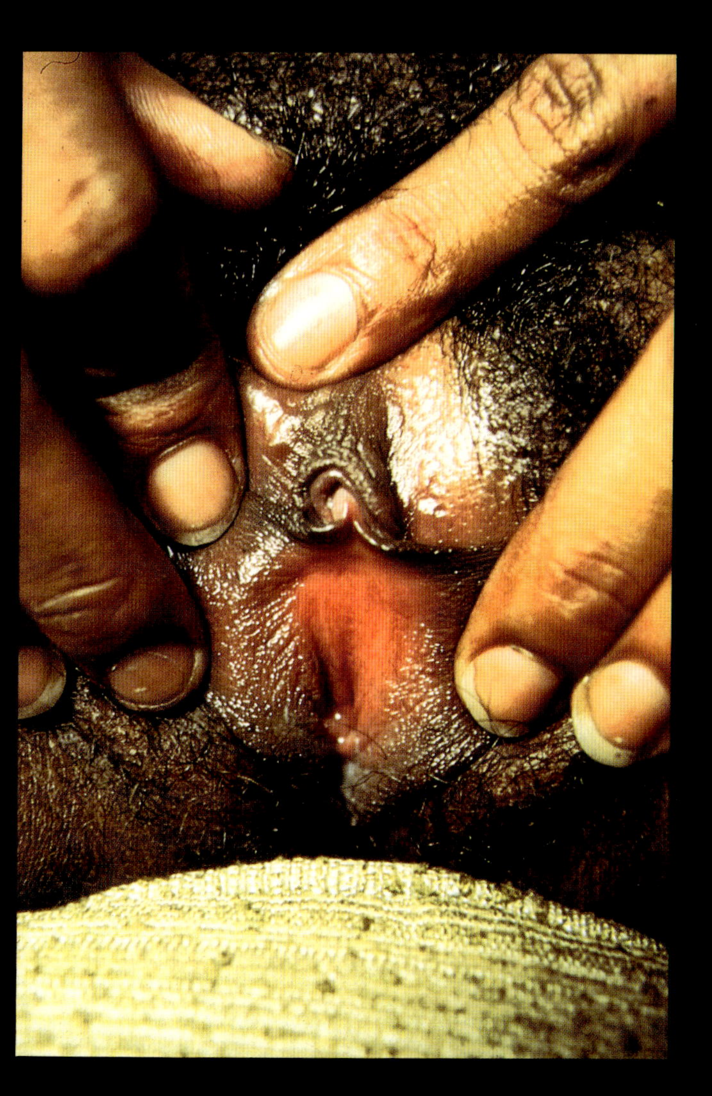

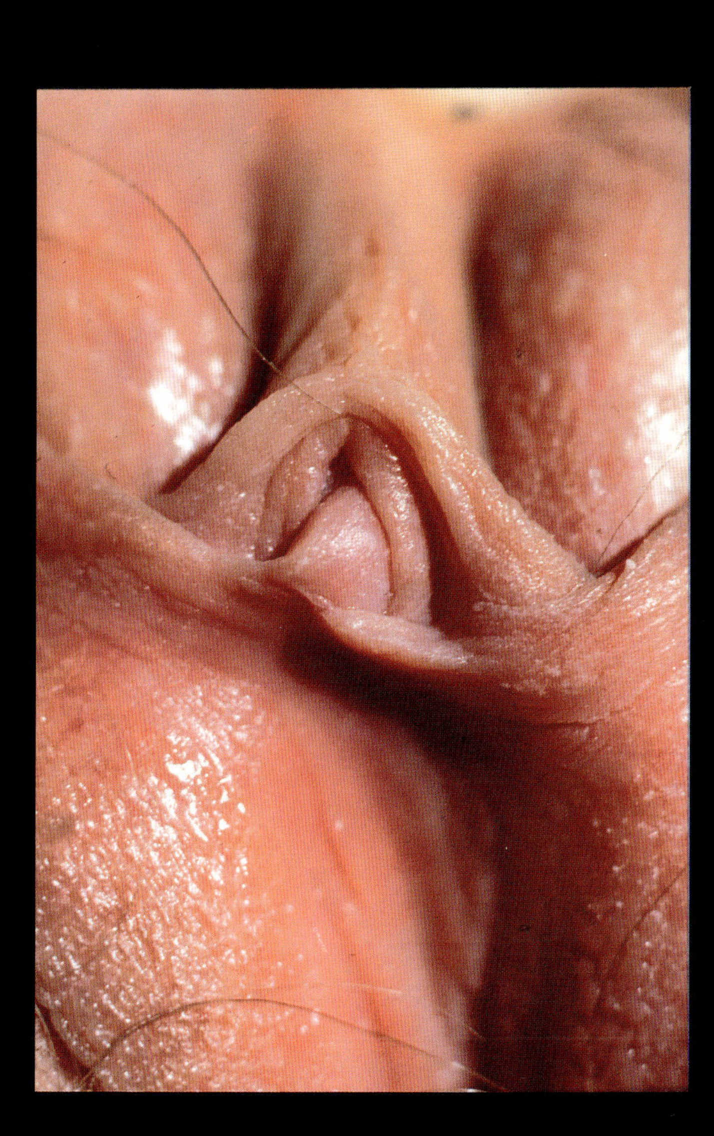

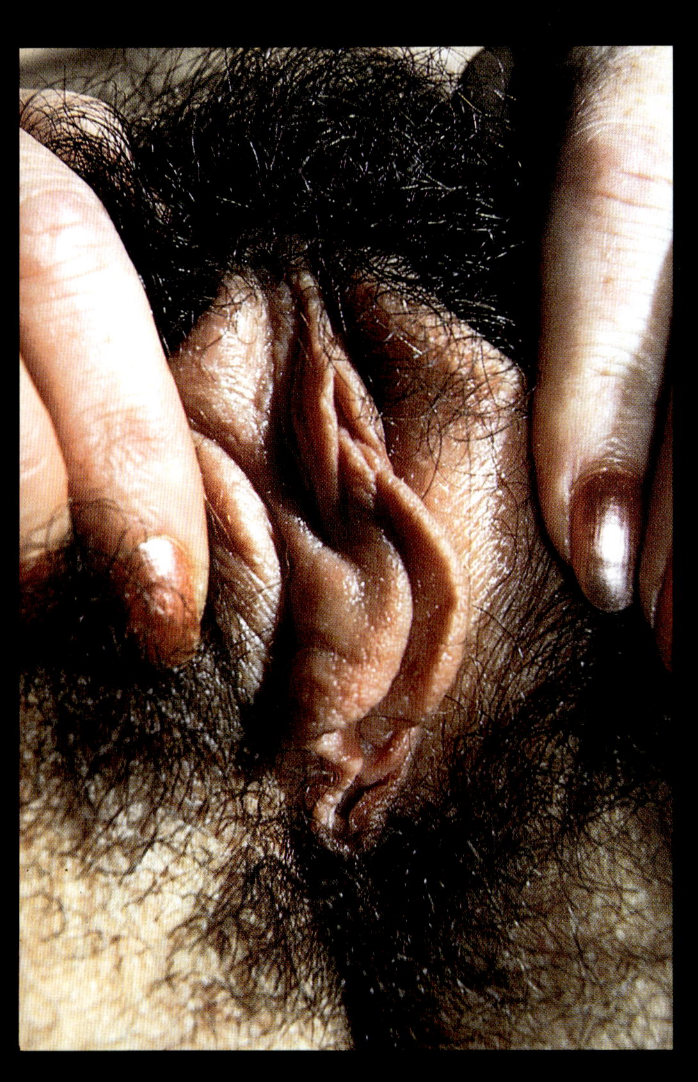

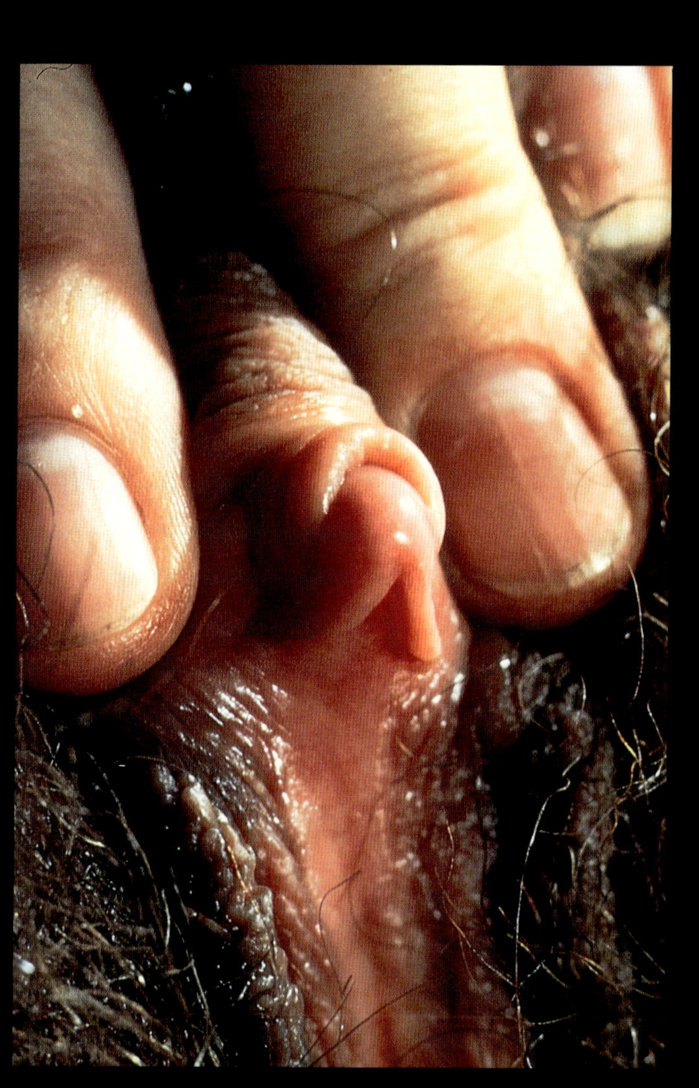

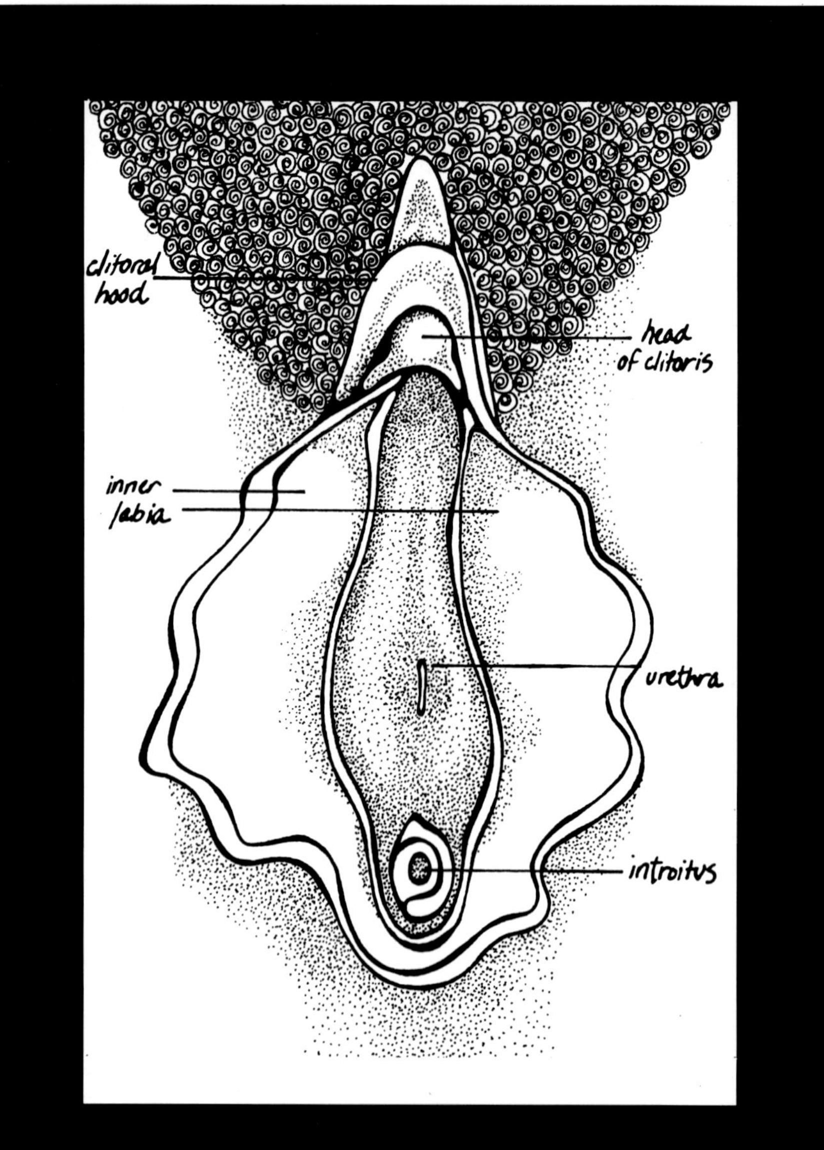
clitoral hood
head of clitoris
inner labia
urethra
introitus

BIBLIOGRAPHY

Becoming Orgasmic, Julia Heiman, Ph.D. and Joseph LoPiccolo, Ph.D. A personal growth program to develop a woman's capacity for arousal and sexual pleasure. Simon & Schuster, 1987.

The Cunt Coloring Book, Tee Corinne. Drawings of women's genitals. Last Gasp, 1988.

Good Vibrations: The Complete Guide to Vibrators, Joani Blank. Everything you wanted to know about vibrators and couldn't imagine asking — where to buy one, how to use one, using one with a partner. Down There Press, 1982, 1989.

Masturbation, Tantra and Self Love, Margo Woods. Down-to-earth discussion of tantric sex. Mho & Mho Works/Omphaloskepsis Press, 1981.

The New Our Bodies, Ourselves, Boston Women's Health Book Collective. An indispensable sourcebook. Simon & Schuster, 1992.

A New View of a Woman's Body, Feminist Women's Health Collective. A feminist self-help classic, with self-exam procedures. Feminist Health Press, 1991.

Ourselves, Growing Older, Paula Brown Doress and Diana Laskin Siegal. Addresses the changing needs of women over thirty-five. Simon & Schuster, 1987.

The Playbook for Women About Sex, Joani Blank. A workbook to enhance sexual awareness. Down There Press, 1975.

Sex for One, Betty Dodson. The premier guide to self-loving. Crown Publishers, Inc., 1987.